~ GOOD MOOD FOODS ~

I0116376

Natural Foods That Support Healthy

Dopamine, Endorphin & Serotonin

Levels in the Body

Rory M. Celmin

Editor: Ginny Greene
Cover Design: Rory M. Celmin

Contact info:
email: RMCBooks@yahoo.com
twitter: @VitalityHealth9

ISBN-13: 978-0-9840186-7-3
ISBN-10: 0984018670

Legal Disclaimer: This book is intended for informational purposes only, is not meant to replace the advice or consultation of a doctor or physician and should not be construed as personal medical advice. Neither the author nor publisher is advocating, offering or participating in any health treatment, professional advice or services to the reader, nor will they be responsible for any adverse effects, damage, injury, loss or consequences allegedly arising from any information, suggestions or recommendations in this book. Readers who fail to consult appropriate health professionals assume the risk of any injuries, and should always consult their doctor or health professional for any matters relating to their health and wellbeing.

~ __Table of Contents__ ~

Hormones & Neurotransmitters 4-5

1. Dopamine 6

2. Foods That Increase Dopamine Levels 7-9

3. Dopamine Foods Chart 10

4. Endorphins 11

5. Foods That Increase Endorphin Levels 12-13

6. Endorphin Foods Chart 14

7. Serotonin 15

8. Foods That Increase Serotonin Levels 16-17

9. Serotonin Foods Chart 18

10. Foods to Avoid 19-20

List of References 21-22

Resourceful Websites 23-24

Nutritional Glossary 25-34

About the Author 35

~ Hormones & Neurotransmitters ~

Believe it or not, certain hormones can actually make us feel happy! These 'feel good' hormones are stimulated by the components of certain foods we eat, and can have a considerable effect on our energy, growth, metabolism, moods, mental focus and sexual reproduction. Understanding the link between our moods and the foods we eat is directly related to how the brain functions.

Both hormones and neurotransmitters are chemicals released inside our brain and play a vital role in many bodily processes. They have a considerable effect on our energy, growth, metabolism, moods, mental focus and sexual reproduction. They share similar traits and are often regarded as the same, but there are several differences between hormones and neurotransmitters.

Hormones are produced by endocrine gland and are directly released into the bloodstream, whereas neurotransmitters are released at nerve synapses (terminals) and are stimulated by an electrical signal. Hormones are secreted slowly, as neurotransmitters are released and act quickly. Hormones can be synthesized from nutrients, but neurotransmitters can only be made inside our body, manufactured from inside the cell of a neuron.

Dopamine, endorphin and serotonin act as both hormones in the bloodstream and neurotransmitters at the nerve terminals. These three are most affected by diet, and are the most influential in effecting mood. Dopamine is associated with feelings of pleasure, motivation, mental alertness and focus. Endorphins are associated with feelings of happiness, euphoria and a lower sensitivity to pain. They are mainly released by exercising, but can also be released by eating certain foods. Serotonin is related to feelings of calm, relaxation, lower levels of stress and anxiety, and having slower reaction time.

Antioxidants, complex carbohydrates and omega 3 fatty acids are the three main groups of nutrition that are responsible for the synthesis of neurotransmitters. Foods such as fruits, vegetables, beans, nuts & seeds and whole grains are rich in antioxidants, vitamins & minerals and fiber that help protect the body from free radicals known to destroy the production of neurotransmitters. Lean protein sources like wild-caught salmon and free-range turkey are both excellent sources of omega-3 fatty acids, and contain some of the highest concentrations of the precursor amino acid *tyrosine,* responsible for the production of neurotransmitters. The following pages detail the relationship between the foods we eat, and the effect hormones and neurotransmitters have on brain function.

~ <u>Dopamine</u> ~

Dopamine is an important chemical messenger manufactured in the brain and adrenal glands. It transmits electric impulses throughout our nervous system, and plays an important role in mood regulation, feelings of pleasure, mental alertness, motivation, gratification and desire. Competitive games, exercise, sexual intercourse, and other gratifying experiences stimulate the release of dopamine. When we've had our fill of dopamine, we experience feelings of pleasure, well-being, mental focus and having well-controlled motor movements.

Acting as a natural antidepressant, dopamine can be released in the body by eating protein-rich foods. The brain needs a constant supply of precursor chemicals that neural cells convert into dopamine. *Tyrosine* is a precursor amino acid that helps the body make two neurotransmitters – dopamine and norepinephrine – that are associated with alertness. Food sources of dopamine-increasing tyrosine include almonds, avocados, bananas, lima beans, fish pumpkin & sesame seeds and watermelon. Foods rich in antioxidants may help protect the production of dopamine from free radical damage.

Dopamine deficiencies are associated with feelings of sadness, depression, lack of motivation and the inability to socialize/love. According to the University of Maryland Medical Center, dopamine deficiency may contribute to physical disorders such as Parkinson's disease and Attention Deficit Hyperactivity Disorder (ADHD), and mood disorders such as depression and chronic boredom.

~ <u>Foods That Increase Dopamine Levels</u> ~

Almonds (raw) ~ contain vitamin B-6 and the amino acid *tyrosine,* both of which help increase dopamine levels in the brain. It promotes the production of new dopamine, as well as another type of neurotransmitter called *norepinephrine*

Apples ~ contain a powerful antioxidant called *quercetin* that protects the body from free radicals that decrease dopamine production and may increase the risk of cancer

Artichokes ~ rich in antioxidants that help eliminate dopamine-lowering free radicals, promotes the production of dopamine

Avocados ~ contain the amino acid tyrosine that helps increase dopamine levels, also a great source of fiber, heart-healthy unsaturated fat, vitamins B6, B9, C, K and potassium that all help generate dopamine in the body

Bananas (ripe) ~ ripe bananas contain high levels of tyrosine which is necessary for dopamine production, and helps increase alertness, concentration, memory and motivation. (the little brown spots on a ripe banana reveal the high concentrations of tyrosine)

Beans/Legumes ~ rich in protein which promotes the production of dopamine, especially lima beans; both beans and legumes form complete proteins when combined with whole grains – providing an excellent source of dopamine-related amino acids

Beets ~ contain the antidepressant amino acid called *betaine* that helps stimulate the production of SAM-e (S-adenoslmethionine) – a nutrient manufactured by the liver which is necessary for the production of dopamine and elevated moods

Bell Peppers ~ trigger dopamine release in the body, rich in vitamin A & C which promotes dopamine synthesis

Berries (blueberries, strawberries) ~ contain high levels of powerful antioxidants that help eliminate free radicals and stimulate the release of dopamine, studies show blueberries most effective

Carrots ~ rich in antioxidants like vitamins A & E which help promote the synthesis of dopamine

Chicken ~ a complete protein that contains all essential amino acids and helps increase dopamine levels, also a great source of the powerful antioxidant coenzyme Q10 (CoQ10) which promotes dopamine production

Citrus Fruits (grapefruits, lemons, oranges) ~ these citrus fruits are rich in antioxidants that support dopamine production and protect our cells from free radical damage

Cottage Cheese ~ a healthy, low-fat substitute for hard/soft cheeses and other dairy products. It contains all nine of the essential amino acids as well as the nonessential amino acids. The protein in cottage cheese helps produce dopamine and norepinephrine in the body, boosting mood and increasing energy levels. (One cup of low-fat cottage cheese provides 28 grams of protein, 2 grams of leucine, 2 grams of lysine and other various amino acids)

Eggs ~ contain all essential amino acids, increases dopamine in the body, protein-rich foods like eggs acts as natural antidepressant

Salmon (wild-caught) ~ ideal source for Omega-3's that increase receptors for dopamine in the brain, contains one of the highest concentrations of tyrosine that support dopamine production (bass, halibut, mackerel, trout, tuna & sardines also great sources of protein)

Seeds (pumpkin, sesame, sunflower) ~ healthful snack rich in vitamins, minerals & amino acids that promote dopamine production

Sweet Potatoes ~ nutrient-rich, complex carbohydrate loaded with antioxidants like vitamin A & C which help promote the synthesis of dopamine (vitamin A deficiencies are associated with low levels of dopamine)

Turkey ~ contains the highest concentration of precursor amino acid *tyrosine* similar to salmon, skinless turkey is healthiest option

Watermelon ~ a tasty fat-free fruit loaded with vitamin B-6 which is needed to manufacture dopamine, also contains high levels of vitamin's A & C which strengthen the immune system while protecting the body from free radical damage that destroys the body's ability to create dopamine

Wheat Germ ~ a great source of vitamin B6 which increases dopamine production, contains the amino acid *phenylalanine* which can convert in the body to tyrosine which is then used to create dopamine

Dopamine Foods Chart

Almonds	Chicken
Apples	Citrus Fruits (grapefruits, lemons, oranges)
Artichokes	Cottage Cheese
Avocados	Eggs
Bananas (ripe)	Salmon
Beans/Legumes	Seeds (pumpkin, sesame, sunflower)
Beets	Sweet Potatoes
Bell Peppers	Turkey
Berries (blueberries, strawberries)	Watermelon
Carrots	Wheat Germ

~ <u>Endorphins</u> ~

Endorphins are 'feel good' hormones that stimulate feelings of bliss and euphoria, reduce anxiety and lower sensitivity to pain. Produced by the pituitary gland, endorphins are released during strenuous exercise and are considered a natural pain reliever. This is what many athletes refer to as the "runners high" – the euphoric feeling that occurs after long, high-intensity workouts cross a threshold and stimulate endorphin production. Cardiovascular, stretching and weight-lifting for over 30 minutes is the most effective way to activate endorphin production through physical exertion and transmit electrical signals throughout the nervous system. Other ways to promote endorphin production include laughing, acupuncture, meditation, massage, having sex and being outdoors in the sunlight.

There are also certain types of natural foods that can help elevate our blissful and euphoric feelings. Eating chocolate helps release endorphins, as well as spicy foods such as chili peppers, jalapenos turmeric and wasabi. Low endorphin levels are may result in low mood swings, and are associated with nutrient deficiencies including vitamins B & C, and the minerals iron, potassium and zinc.

~ Foods That Increase Endorphin Levels ~

Bananas ~ contain the mineral potassium which is necessary for nerve function, provide an energy-packed carbohydrate which helps sustain good moods and keep you feeling energetic

Brown rice ~ great source of complex carbohydrates, fiber and B vitamins which increase endorphin levels

Chili Peppers (cayenne pepper) ~ cause the body to release endorphins to help alleviate the heat these peppers produce; the hotter the pepper – the more endorphins are released

Chocolate (dark) ~ contains high quantities of antioxidants and polyphenols which boost mood, produce euphoric feelings and heighten sensitivity, also contains *phenylethylamine* – a substance associated with infatuation, love and sexual attraction

Grapes ~ great source of endorphin-producing vitamin C and endorphin-releasing potassium, also rich in powerful antioxidants called *polyphenols*

Horseradish ~ a spicy condiment that stimulates the production and release of endorphins in the body

Jalapenos ~ like hot peppers, are among the most effective spicy foods for stimulating the production and release of endorphins...ole!

Nuts ~ great source of B vitamins and protein, rich in the mineral selenium which contain mood-enhancing properties (Brazil nuts contain the most selenium), also great source of unsaturated fats

Citrus Fruits (lemons, limes, oranges) ~ excellent source of vitamin C which helps increase the production of endorphins, also rich in B vitamins and a powerful type of antioxidant called *flavonoids*

Pasta (whole grain) ~ great source of non-fat protein, contains amino acids *L-phenylalanine* & *tryptophan* which help stimulate endorphin production, also rich in dietary fiber & B vitamins (a lack of protein in the diet is associated with depressed moods)

Sesame Seeds ~ great source of protein and powerful antioxidants such as vitamins E, also rich in B vitamins, calcium, iron & magnesium

Strawberries ~ rich in vitamin C which increases endorphin production, contains potassium which assists in the generation and transport of nerve impulses throughout our central nervous system, also contains a powerful antioxidant called *anthocyanin*

Turmeric ~ bright yellow spice used in curry and mustards that stimulates the production of endorphins, excellent source of antioxidants and is known to be a powerful aphrodisiac

Wasabi ~ Asian sushi spice that helps releases endorphins from the brain to the rest o the body

Endorphin Foods Chart

Bananas	Nuts
Brown Rice	Oranges
Chili Peppers	Pasta (whole grain)
Chocolate (dark)	Sesame Seeds
Grapes	Strawberries
Horseradish	Turmeric
Jalapenos	Wasabi

~ <u>Serotonin</u> ~

Serotonin is known as the 'happiness' hormone because it is responsible for regulating moods and making you feel happy. This neurotransmitter is also known for affecting appetite, sleep patterns, learning and memory. Serotonin can be released in the body by exposure to sunlight, laughing and exercising and getting a restful night's sleep.

Amino acids, vitamins and minerals are necessary for serotonin production. Serotonin cannot be produced in the body without the amino acid *tryptophan*. When tryptophan-rich protein is consumed with low-glycemic complex carbohydrates, tryptophan is able to cross the blood-brain barrier and form serotonin. Having a turkey and cranberry sandwich on whole grain bread, or chicken and brown rice are great ways to elevate your serotonin levels. Essential fatty acids EPA & DHA from sources like wild-caught salmon contain tryptophan and are necessary for serotonin production and elevated moods. Foods rich in B6 increase serotonin levels. Vitamin B9 (folic acid) and vitamin B12 work synergistically to produce serotonin, and vitamin C assists in increasing serotonin levels as well.

Nettle tea is a great source of vitamins, minerals and flavonoids which has been used to increase serotonin levels. The nutritional supplements St John's Wort and 5-HTP are also known or stimulating serotonin production. Serotonin can be replenished after a restful night sleep; however if sleep is missed, serotonin levels are depleted the next day leaving one feeling tired with low energy and deflated moods. A lack of tryptophan is associated with anxiety, feeling low, mood disorders, sugar cravings and irritable bowel syndrome (IBS).

~ Foods That Increase Serotonin Levels ~

Asparagus ~ a delicious health food rich in antioxidants and nutrients that increase serotonin levels in the body

Avocados ~ contain monounsaturated fats and essential fatty acids which increase serotonin levels and normalize hormonal processes

Bananas (ripe) ~ excellent source of tryptophan, vitamin B6 and healthful carbohydrates that increase levels of serotonin in the body, ideal when combined with whey protein (in a shake) and provide vital post-workout nutrition that restores electrolytes lost during exercise

Beans ~ a nutrient-dense complex carbohydrate with a low glycemic index (GI) that helps raise serotonin levels

Beets ~ contain the amino acid called *betaine* (known as an antidepressant) that helps stimulate the production of SAM-e (S-adenosylmethionine) – a nutrient manufactured by the liver which is necessary for the production of serotonin and elevated moods

Cherries (sour) ~ contain melatonin which is necessary for sleeping well, and a restful night's sleep helps replenish serotonin levels

Chicken ~ excellent source of vitamin B6 and tryptophan which are both important for raising serotonin levels in the brain

Chocolate (dark) ~ rich in antioxidants and polyphenols, is well known to increase serotonin levels in the brain (just don't eat too much at one time – when your blood sugar crashes your serotonin levels will also drop – moderation is important!)

Eggs ~ excellent source of protein, contain amino acids and essential fatty acids EPA and DHA which are necessary for serotonin production (especially egg whites)

Nuts (pecans, walnuts) ~ great source of protein and dietary fiber, nuts are rich in tryptophan which increases serotonin levels and help maintain elevated moods

Pineapples ~ contain vitamins, minerals, enzymes and significant amounts of tryptophan required for serotonin production

Salmon (wild caught) ~ rich in omega 3 essential fatty acids DHA & EPA as well as tryptophan – both necessary for the production of serotonin, maintaining elevated moods & maintaining thyroid health

Sunflowers Seeds (raw) ~ an excellent source of the amino acid tryptophan that converts to serotonin in the brain

Sweet Potatoes ~ a nutrient-dense complex carbohydrate loaded with B vitamins and tryptophan which increase serotonin levels

Turkey (free range) ~ excellent source of protein rich in tryptophan – an amino acid necessary for maintaining healthy serotonin levels

Whey protein ~ one of the best sources of protein that increases serotonin levels, also regulates appetite, helps control blood sugar levels and boosts the immune system

Whole Grains (brown rice, buckwheat, flax, oats) ~ low-glycemic complex carbohydrates contain both tryptophan and high levels of omega 3 fatty acids which are great for raising serotonin levels, they are also rich in vitamin B6 necessary for proper serotonin synthesis in the brain as well as increased energy levels and elevated moods

Yogurt ~ excellent source of vegetarian protein, rich in the amino acid tryptophan that increase serotonin levels in the body (adding fruit to yogurt further boosts serotonin levels)

Serotonin Foods Chart

Asparagus	Nuts (pecans, walnuts)
Avocados	Pineapples
Bananas	Salmon
Beans	Sunflower Seeds
Beets	Sweet Potatoes
Cherries (tart)	Turkey
Chicken	Whey Protein
Chocolate (dark)	Whole Grains (buckwheat, flax, oat)
Eggs	Yogurt

~ **Foods to Avoid** ~

The foods we eat and our eating habits are directly related to our moods, energy level and mental focus. Eating organic vegetables, fresh fruits, lean protein and other nutrient-dense foods will help normalize hormonal functions, increase energy levels and keep us feeling happier. Fats from healthy sources such as wild-caught salmon, real butter (in moderation), coconut oil and olive oil are also a great option.

Foods high in cholesterol, sugar and saturated fats may provide a temporary feeling of satisfaction, but they interfere with proper brain function and eventually deplete our 'feel good' hormones. Hormone imbalance is associated with fatigue, insomnia, low libido, mood swings, weight gain and many other disorders that can significantly lessen the quality of life. The following page lists types of foods and lifestyle habits that should be **avoided** to help maintain proper health and hormone balance.

Alcohol ~ powerful sedative that causes dehydration, alcohol should be avoided by those with hormonal imbalances

Caffeine ~ should be avoided by those with depression or hormonal imbalances, caffeine is a stimulant and temporarily elevates mood and increases serotonin levels, but decreases after the 'caffeine crash'

Large Meals ~ a fully belly keeps food in the stomach longer, diverting blood to the stomach for digestion and away from the brain, muscles and other organs which makes us feel tired

Excessive Carbohydrates ~ simple carbohydrates like potato chips, table sugar and white bread cause a spike in blood sugar which is temporarily satisfying, but soon causes a blood sugar crash which depletes dopamine as well as energy levels

Omega-6 Polyunsaturated Fats ~ avoid canola, peanut, vegetable and soybean oils, as well as margarine, shortening and other synthetic fats

Plastic Cookware/Storage ~ avoid heating or storing foods in plastic – cook in glass or non-coated metal pans

Sleep (lack of) ~ may lead to a hormonal imbalance, also associated with a shortened life, increased susceptibility to disease and obesity

Toxins ~ found in household chemicals, cleaners, foods, pesticides, plastics, they mimic hormones in the body while inhibiting our body's ability to produce real hormones

~ List of References ~

*Anderson, Jean E. M.S., Deskins, Barbara Ph.D. *The Nutrition Bible – A Comprehensive No-Nonsense Guide to Foods, Nutrients, Additives, Preservatives, Pollutants and Everything Else We Eat and Drink.* New York, NY: HarperCollins Publishers, 1997

*Balch, Phyllis A., CNC. *Prescription for Nutritional Healing, 5th edition.* New York, NY: Penguin Group (Avery), 2010

*Beck, Leslie R.D. *Leslie Beck's Nutrition Encyclopedia.* Toronto, Ontario: Penguin Group, 2003

*Clements, Ed. *Ten Delicious Bodybuilding Foods That Increase Serotonin Levels.* Muscle-Health-Fitness, December 14, 2012

*Dunlop BW, Nemeroff CB. *The Role of Dopamine in the Pathophysiology of Depression.* Arch Gen Psychiatry. 2007

*Hart, Gillian R., M.D. *The biological role of Vitamin D and Methods for Measurement. CLI,* ImmunoDiagnostic Systems (IDS), Inc. Sept. 2005

*Jacka, Felice. *Association of Western and Traditional Diets with Depression and Anxiety in Women.* The American Journal of Psychiatry, January 4, 2010;167:305-311

*Kirschmann, Gayla J. and Kirschmann, John D. *Nutrition Almanac, 4th edition.* New York, NY: McGraw-Hill, 1996

*Konlee, Mark & LeBeau Conrad *Immune Restoration Handbook, 2nd edition.*Keep Hope Alive, Ltd, 2004

*Mark, Margery H., M.D. *Parkinson's Disease: Pathogenesis, Diagnosis and Treatment.* Dept. of Neurology, UNDMJ-Robert Woodsen Johnson Medical School, 2005

*Praschak-Rieder, Nicole M.D. *Seasonal Variation in Human Brain Serotonin Transporter Binding.* Archives of General Psychiatry, September 2008;65(9):1072-1078

*Price, Weston A., D.D.S. *Nutrition and Physical Degeneration, 8th edition.* San Diego, CA: Price-Pottenger Nutrition Foundation, 2008

*Robinson, Donald S., M.D. *The Role of Dopamine and Norepinephrine in Depression,* Burlington, VT: Primary Psychiatry, 2007

*Roizen, Michael F., M.D. and Oz, Mehmet C., M.D. *You Staying Young – The Owners Manual for Extending Your Warranty.* New York, NY: Free Press, 2007

*Schneier, Franklin R. M.D. *Social Anxiety Disorder.* New England Journal of Medicine, 2006 Sept 7;355(10):1029-36.

*Somer, Elizabeth M.A., R.D. *Food & Mood – The Complete Guide to Eating Well and Feeling Your Best, 2nd edition.* New York, NY: Owl Books, 1999

*Tessmer, Kimberly A. R.D., L.D. *The Everything Nutrition Book – Boost Energy, Prevent Illness and Live Longer.* Avon, MA: Adams Media, 2003

*Trattler, Ross N.D., D.O. and Jones, Adrian N.D. *Better Health Through Natural Healing, 2nd edition.* Heatherton VIC, Australia: Hinkler Books, 2001

*Trowell, Hubert C. and Burkitt, Denis P. *Western Diseases: Their Emergence and Prevention.* Cambridge, MA: Harvard University Press, 1981

*Wilson, Dr. Lawrence. *Legal Guidelines for Unlicensed Practitioners.* Prescott, AZ: L.D. Wilson Consultants, 2007

~ **Resourceful Websites** ~

American Journal of Psychiatry ~ ajp.psychiatryonline.org

American Society for Nutrition (ASN) – www.nutrition.org

Columbia University Medical Center – www.cumc.columbia.edu

EnCognitive – www.encognitive.com

Hippocrates Health Institute (HHI) – www.hippocratesinst.org

ImmunoDiagnostic Systems (IDS) – www.idsplc.com

Institute of Food Technologists (IFT) – www.ift.org

Institute for Optimum Nutrition – www.ion.ac.uk

Integrative Psychiatry Inc. – www.integrativepsychiatry.net

Live Strong Foundation – www.livestrong.com

Linus Pauling Institute-Oregon State University – www.lpi.oregonstate.edu

Medical News Today – www.medicalnewstoday.com

Medicine Plus (US Nat. Library of Medicine) – www.nlm.nih.gov/medicineplus

Mental Health America (MHA) – www.nmha.org

National Academy of Sciences (NAS) – www.nationalacademies.org

National Center for Complementary and Alternative Medicine (NCCAM) – www.nccam.nih.gov

National Institutes of Health – www.nih.gov

Natural Health Research Institute (NHRI) – www.naturalhealthresearch.org

Neurology Channel – www.neurologychannel.com

The Neurosciences Institute – www.nsi.edu

New England Journal of Medicine – www.nejm.org

Nutrition.gov – www.nutrition.gov

The Nutrition Society – www.nutritionsociety.org

Oasis Advanced Wellness – www.oasisadvancedwellness.com

Organic Authority – www.organicauthority.com

The Organic Center – www.organic-center.org

Organic Consumers Association (OCA) – www.organicconsumers.org

Organic Trade Association (OTA) – www.ota.com

Precision Nutrition – www.precisionnutrition.com

Primary Psychiatry – www.primarypsychiatry.com

University Health Services (UC Berkeley) – www.uhs.berkeley.edu

University of Maryland Medical Center – www.umm.edu

WebMD – www.webmd.com

Whole Foods Market – www.wholefoodsmarket.com

~ Nutritional Glossary ~

A

Absorption – process of assimilating nutrients into the body

Adaptogen – herbal substances that reduce stress and promote beneficial adjustments in the body

Alpha-carotene – phytonutrient found in carrots beneficial for eye health

Alpha-linolenic acid (ALA) – omega-3 essential fatty acid found in flaxseed, pumpkin & soybean oils

Amino acid – nitrogen and carbon-based compounds that build protein and muscle

Anabolic – substance that helps convert nutrition into building and repairing muscle tissues in the body

Antacid – substance that neutralizes stomach acid

Antibody – immune system protein that combats bacteria, fungus and other foreign substances

Antigen – substance that provokes the creation of antibodies

Antihistamine – substance that binds with histamine receptors and reduces the effects of histamines

Antioxidant – substance that minimizes free radical damage to the heart, arteries, and tissues, such as vitamins, minerals and nutrients

Arachidonic acid (AA) – omega-6 essential fatty acid found in eggs, meat, poultry and shellfish

Ascorbic acid – organic compound known as vitamin C

B

Beta carotene – phytonutrient with antioxidant properties the body uses to produce vitamin A, found in broccoli, carrots, collard greens, kale, pumpkin, spinach and sweet potatoes

Bio-availability – ease of which nutrients can be absorbed into the body

Bioflavonoid – group of substances essential for the absorption of vitamin C

Blood sugar – concentration of glucose in the blood

C

Carbohydrate – organic substance that is our main source of energy

Carcinogen – toxic substance capable of producing cancer

Carotene – substance that is converted into vitamin A in the body

Cartenoids – phytonutrients that contain antioxidant properties

Cellulose – organic carbohydrate from fruits and vegetables

Chelation – chemical process where molecules bind to a mineral atom increasing its bio-availability

Chelation therapy – introduction of substances into the body to remove heavy metals

Chlorophyll – green pigment in plants that is vital for photosynthesis; converting light into energy

Cholesterol – steroid metabolite compound including lipids (fats) naturally produced by the body, a structural component of cell membranes, helps absorption of fatty acids; HDL (good) and LDL (bad)

Citric acid – organic acid found in citrus fruits

Coenzyme – substance that works with enzymes to promote normal enzyme activity

Complete protein – protein that contains all 8 essential amino acids

Complex carbohydrate – carbohydrate that provides fiber and slowly releases sugar into the body

Conjugated Linoleic Acid (CLA) – naturally occurring fatty-acid that helps reduce body fat

Cordyceps – rare medicinal mushroom used in Traditional Chinese Medicine for over 5,000 years to strengthen the immune system, improve adrenal function, lower blood pressure and cholesterol, prevent kidney disease and liver disorders

Cortisol – one of the main catabolic hormones in the body

Creatine – high-energy compound in muscle cells which stores energy and increases strength

Cruciferous – 'cross-shaped' blossoms that support digestive health (broccoli, cabbage, cauliflower)

D

Detoxification – process of eliminating toxic substances from the body

Diuretic – substance that increases urine flow

Docosahexaenoic acid (DHA) – omega-3 essential fatty acid found in marine micro-algae, anchovies, cod, mackerel, salmon and tuna

E

Eicosapentaenoic acid (EPA) – omega-3 essential fatty acid found in cod, salmon, sardines and tuna

Electrolytes (potassium, sodium and chloride) – soluble substances containing free ions capable of conducting electric impulses throughout the body

Enzyme – protein catalyst that manages chemical reactions in the body

Essential Fatty Acids (EFA's) – amino acids that cannot be synthesized by the body and must be supplied by foods or supplements

F

Fat-soluble – ability to dissolve in fats and oils

Fatty acid – carboxylic acid derived from natural fats and oils

Fiber – indigestible plant matter that helps eliminate toxins from the body (fruits, vegetables, nuts, legumes, whole grains)

Flavonoid – class of substances found in plants that help protect against cancer

Fructose – sugar found in fruit that has a low glycemic index

G

Gamma-linolenic acid (GLA) – omega-6 essential fatty acid found in borage & primrose oil

Gland – organ that synthesizes substances for release into the bloodstream

Glucose – simple sugar in the blood that is the major energy source for the body's cells and functions

Gluten – protein found in oats, wheat, barley and rye

Glycemic Index (GI) – measure of how much food raises blood sugar levels as compared to white bread, which has a GI of 100 (the lower the number the less insulin is released by the body)

Glycogen – the main form of glucose stored in the body, then converts back to glucose to supply energy

Growth Hormone (GH) – hormone that is released by the pituitary gland that promotes muscle growth and the breakdown of body fat for energy

H

HDL cholesterol (high-density lipoprotein) – known as *good cholesterol*, helps clear fat from bloodstream and indicates low risk of cardiovascular disease

Heavy metals (arsenic, cadmium, lead, mercury) – elements that possess metallic properties and have a gravity measurement greater than 5.0

Herbal therapy – herbal combination of tinctures, extracts and capsules used for cleansing and healing

Histamine – chemical released by the immune system that has potential negative effects on the body

Homeopathy – alternative medicines using herbs, natural substances to strengthen the immune system

Hormone – vital substance produced by body to regulate biological processes

Hydrochloric acid (HCL) – strong corrosive stomach acid that helps digestion

Hydrogenation – process by which hydrogen atoms are combined with oil molecules to turn liquid oils into solids, destroying nutritional value of the oil

Hypoallergenic – having a low capacity for being affected by allergies

I

Immune system – complex system of organs, cells and proteins that protect the body against disease

Inorganic – substances that do not contain carbon

Insulin – anabolic hormone produced by pancreas that regulates blood sugar

Intestinal flora – friendly bacteria in the digestive tract that are essential for digestion and metabolism

Isoflavones – class of phytonutrients that protect against estrogen-based cancers like breast cancer

K

Kefir – fermented milk product that contains anti-aging properties

Ketosis – process of metabolism where the liver converts fats into fatty acids and is used for energy

Kombucha – sweetened fermented tea beverage that has detoxifying effects and healing properties

L

Lactase – enzyme that converts lactose into glucose and is necessary for digesting milk and dairy

Lactic acid – acid created from glucose metabolism that accumulates in the body after strenuous exercise causing muscle fatigue and pain

Lactose – term referring to milk sugar

Lauric acid – fatty acid found in coconut and palm kernel oil that has antimicrobial properties

LDL cholesterol (low density lipoprotein) – known as *bad cholesterol,* associated with increased risk of cardiovascular disease

Legumes (alfalfa, beans, carob, lentils, peanuts, peas, soy) – seed pod that splits both sides when ripe

Lentils (beluga, black, green, red, white, yellow) – leguminous, climbing-vine plant containing only 2 seeds to a pod

Liminoids – phytonutrients found in citrus fruits that help inhibit the production of cancer cells and HIV protease activity

Linolenic acid (LA) – omega-6 essential fatty acid found in corn oil, safflower and sunflower oil

Lipids – natural substances that are soluble in the same solvents as fats and oils

Lipolysis – refers to the chemical breakdown of body fat by enzymes that produce energy

Lipoprotein – protein molecule that helps transport fats around the bloodstream

Lipotropic – substances that breaks down fat and helps manage blood sugar

Lutein – phytonutrient that helps protect against macular degeneration (spinach, kale, turnip greens)

Lycopene – phytonutrient that helps protect against prostate cancer and ultraviolet rays from the sun (guava, pink grapefruit, tomatoes and watermelon)

M

Macrobiotics – referring to a branch of Eastern medicine that uses grain as a staple food, and balances Yin (negative) and Yang (positive) foods together to overcome health issues

Macronutrients (proteins, carbohydrates and fats) – essential elements needed in large quantities to sustain proper health

Malabsorption – inability to absorb nutrients from intestines into bloodstream

Metabolism – process by which cells absorb nutrition & change food into energy

Mineral – naturally occurring substance that is essential for human life and vital to metabolic processes

Monounsaturated fats (canola, olive, peanut and sunflower oils) – fatty acids that are not saturated with hydrogen, typically liquid at room temperature but will solidify when refrigerated

N

Naturopathy – alternative form of medicine using a combination of natural methods to combat disease and maintain health

Neurotransmitter – chemical messenger that transmit electric signals from the brain throughout the nervous system

Nonessential Amino Acids – amino acids that can be produced by the body from other amino acids, therefore not essential to the human diet

Nutrient – natural substance all living organisms need for growth and survival

Nutrition – the science of converting food into fuel for the body

O

Organic – referring to foods that are grown naturally, without the use of synthetic chemicals like herbicides, pesticides or hormones

Oxalates (oxalic acid) – organic substances found in humans, plants and animals of which high concentrations may lead to kidney stones; (oxalic acid foods include: amaranth, beans, beet greens, beer, berries, celery, chocolate, figs, kale, kiwi, leeks, nuts/seeds, okra, parsley, plums, quinoa, rhubarb, soy foods, spinach, squash, Swiss chard, tangerines, watercress, wheat germ)

P

pH (potential of hydrogen) – measurement of the acidity and alkalinity of a substance or solution

Photosynthesis – synthesis of organic compounds from inorganic compounds by plants and algae involving light energy

Phytonutrients – natural substances found in fruits and vegetables that protect the body against disease (chlorophyll, carotenoids, flavonoids, isoflavones, inositol, lignans, indoles, phenols, sulfides, terpenes)

Polyphenols – group of compounds found in plants that have at least one phenol unit per molecule

Polysaccharides – class of carbohydrates which breaks down during hydrolysis to a monosaccharide

Probiotics – substances that promote the growth of friendly bacteria in the body

Protein – nitrogen-based compounds made from amino acids that are the basic components of animal and vegetable tissues, needed for growth and repair

Proteolytic enzymes – break down proteins and help reduce the risk of cancer

Purines – natural substances that are part of the chemical structure of human, plant and animal genes, high concentrations may lead to arthritis, gout and inflammation (purine-rich foods include: anchovies, asparagus, bacon, beef, cauliflower, chicken, eggs, ham, herring, mackerel, mushrooms, mussels, oatmeal, organ meats, peas, pork, sardines, shellfish, smelt, spinach, sweetbreads, turkey, yeast),

R

RDA (Recommended Daily Allowance) – basic amount of nutrients that should be consumed daily to maintain proper health

Retinoic acid – acid from vitamin A

S

Saliva – mixture of water, protein and salts making food easy to swallow/digest

Saturated fat (butter, chocolate, dairy, lard, meat) – unhealthy fat, typically solid at room temperature and has been shown to raise cholesterol levels

Simple carbohydrate – carbohydrate quickly absorbed into bloodstream

Stevia – natural herbal sweetener native to South America sweeter than sugar

Sucrose – table sugar

Synergy – harmonious interaction between two or more substances where their combined ability is greater than their individual actions

T

Thermogenics – supplements that increase metabolism and generate heat

Thyroid gland – internal thermostat regulating body temperature by secreting hormones that control energy used and calories burned

Tolerance – capability of an organism to endure an unfavorable environment

Toxin – poison that impairs health and bodily functions

Trace element – mineral required by the body in minute quantities for proper growth and development

Trans-fat – unsaturated fat produced through hydrogenation; increases risk of cardiovascular disease

Triglyceride – compound made up of three fatty acids and glycerol and is how fat is stored in the body

U

Unsaturated fat (olive, flaxseed, safflower and fish oils) – known as healthy fat, helps reduce cholesterol and triglycerides levels in the blood

V

Vitamin – organic substance obtained through diet to maintain proper health and support many biological functions

W

Water-soluble – ability to dissolve in water

X

Xylitol – natural sweetener made from birch bark that has antifungal properties, has a low glycemic index (GI) score and alkalizes the body

Y

Yang (heat, light and dryness) – one of two essential principles of Chinese medicine needed to create balance and harmony in the body, organs include the gallbladder, spleen, intestines and skin

Yin (cold, shadow and moisture) – the other essential principle of Chinese medicine needed to create balance and harmony in the body, organs include the liver, heart, kidneys, lungs and bones

Z

Zeaxanthin – phytonutrient that protects against macular degeneration found in citrus fruits, eggs and green vegetables

~ **About the Author** ~

Rory M. Celmin is certified in sports nutrition from the International Fitness Professional Association (IFPA), received a Bachelor's Degree in English from California State University San Marcos (CSUSM) and has studied health and nutrition for over 20 years. He is the author of *Nature's Nutrition – A Comprehensive Resource Guide for Super Foods, Natural Supplements and Preventative Health*, which was named Finalist in the "Diet/Nutrition/Food" category of the 2012 Next Generation Indie Book Awards, and received Honorable Mention in the "How To" category of the 2012 Beach Book Festival. Rory is a Nutrition Coach at "Natural Advantage Nutritional Consulting" and in his spare time enjoys tennis, basketball, surfing, hiking and photography, and resides in sunny California.

Contact: RMCBooks@yahoo.com

Twitter: @VitalityHealth9

www.ingramcontent.com/pod-product-compliance
Lightning Source LLC
Chambersburg PA
CBHW041223270326
41933CB00001B/25